Understanding

GW01003747

CHOLE_____
& HEART DISEASE

Professor Barry Lewis

Published by Family Doctor Publications Limited
in association with the British Medical Association

IMPORTANT

This book is intended to supplement the advice given to you by your doctor. The author and publisher have taken every care in its preparation. In particular, information about drugs and dosages has been thoroughly checked. However, before taking any medication you are strongly advised to read the product information sheet accompanying it. Your pharmacist will be able to help you with anything you do not understand.

© Family Doctor Publications 1993, 1995
Reprinted 1994
Second edition 1995

Medical Editor: Dr Tony Smith
Cover Artist: Colette Blanchard
Medical Artist: Angela Christie
Design: Fox Editorial, Guildford, Surrey
Printing: Reflex Litho Ltd, using acid-free paper

ISBN: 1 898205 03 5

Contents

Introduction

The heart is a muscular pump that works day and night, from birth to death. But it can go wrong and one of the commonest forms of heart disease is a heart attack. A heart attack is the result of a blockage or narrowing of one of the coronary arteries (or one of their branches) that supply blood to the heart muscle. This process of arterial narrowing causes coronary heart disease, and it is very common.

In 1992, 170,000 people in Britain died from coronary heart disease, making it a greater killer than cancer.

In 1992, 170,000 people in Britain died from coronary heart disease, making it a greater killer than cancer

Risk factors

Anything about you that increases your chances of getting coronary heart disease, such as smoking, obesity and high blood pressure, is called a risk factor. These are discussed in this book, but it concentrates mainly on one risk factor, the amount of cholesterol in the blood. The risks of smoking and high blood pressure are now widely recognized, but although cholesterol plays a major role in arterial narrowing, many of us are unsure about what it is, what it does and what steps we can take to keep our level of cholesterol within safe limits.

Prevention is better than cure

Coronary heart disease is a serious condition; although it can often be improved by treatment it cannot be cured. Prevention has to be the main goal and so it is vitally important that we all know what we can do to reduce our chances of developing heart trouble.

Cross-section of the heart.

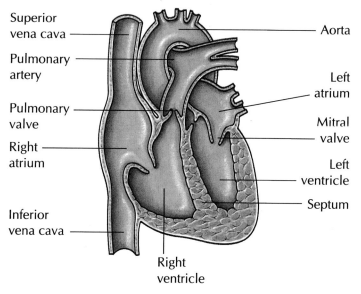

Superior vena cava

Pulmonary artery

Pulmonary valve

Right atrium

Inferior vena cava

Right ventricle

Aorta

Left atrium

Mitral valve

Left ventricle

Septum

The coronary arteries supply blood to the muscles of the heart.

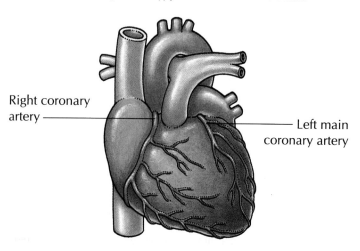

Right coronary artery

Left main coronary artery

What goes wrong

The heart

The function of the heart is to maintain the circulation of the blood by pumping it around the body. Its thick, muscular walls enclose four chambers, the right and left atria (single: atrium) and the right and left ventricles. The right and left sides of the heart are separated from each other by the septa (single: septum), and valves ensure that blood flows only one way. The main arteries carry blood from the left ventricle to all parts of the body with each heart beat; the main veins return blood from the rest of the body to the right atrium.

Arteries and veins

The blood in the arteries carries oxygen and nourishment to all the tissues of the body. Arteries have thick walls because blood is pumped along them under high pressure. Veins carry blood containing carbon dioxide and waste products away from the body tissues. Veins have valves that stop the blood flowing in the wrong direction.

The circulation

Because the tissues of the body use up oxygen, the blood that returns from the body to the right side of the heart is relatively low in oxygen and high in carbon dioxide. The heart pumps this blood through the lungs. There it absorbs oxygen and gets rid of waste carbon dioxide, which is breathed out. The oxygenated blood then returns to the left side of the heart, from where it is pumped through the aorta (main artery) to all parts of the body. The health of every organ in the body requires the heart to pump efficiently, so enabling the arteries to carry the oxygenated blood normally.

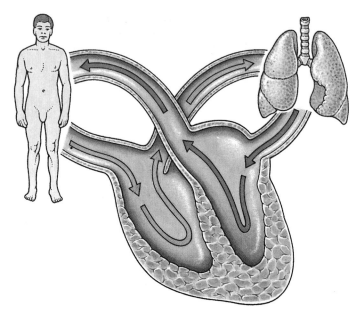

The heart is a pump that circulates blood round the body. Blood from which some of the oxygen has been used (shown in blue) is pumped from the right ventricle into the lungs. Here waste carbon dioxide is breathed out and oxygen is absorbed from the air breathed in. The oxygenated blood (red) returns to the left ventricle, from where it is pumped to all parts of the body.

What happens in a heart attack?

The heart, like other parts of the body, needs oxygen and nutrients and, because it has to work continuously, it requires a generous flow of oxygenated blood. This is delivered through the coronary arteries. When a branch of a coronary artery becomes blocked, the part of the heart wall that was previously supplied with blood from that branch is damaged, some of it irreversibly. Part of the muscle in the region that has been deprived of oxygen dies (a process called myocardial infarction), and in the following weeks the dead muscle is replaced by scar tissue. Unlike heart muscle, this scar tissue cannot contract, so if the area of dead tissue is large or if the person has had a number of heart attacks, the heart becomes a less efficient pump. If severe enough, this can be fatal.

The main symptom of a heart attack is pain. This is felt in the chest, arms, throat or jaw, and usually lasts for about an hour or

FORMS OF CORONARY HEART DISEASE

Typically, coronary heart disease shows itself in one of three ways:

- a heart attack, caused by blocking of a coronary artery branch, which damages the heart muscle;
- angina pectoris, brief attacks of pain on exertion or stress;
- sudden, fatal failure of the heart due to a blocked coronary artery which leads to a seriously abnormal heart rhythm.

severe, but it may be mild. Heart attacks can be painless and 'silent', especially in older people. The main danger, particularly in the first hours, is that the pumping of blood lessens or almost stops, mostly because of irregularities in the heart beat or simply through weakness of the pumping action. If the patient is in hospital, changes in the rhythm and strength of the heart's pumping action can be seen early and can usually be treated.

Angina pectoris

Another symptom of coronary heart disease is called angina pectoris. In angina, brief attacks of pain occur, usually during exercise, and go away at rest. These attacks are more likely to happen in cold

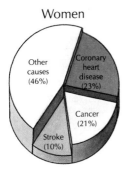

Women

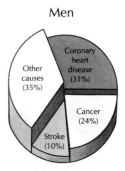

Men

Coronary heart disease is a major cause of death in Britain.

until treatment is given. With the pain may come sweating, shortness of breath or collapse. Typically, the pain starts quite suddenly and is

weather and after a heavy meal. Angina happens because a coronary artery is narrowed to the extent that it allows enough blood through to nourish the heart while resting, but not enough to cope with the demand for more oxygen during exercise. The narrowing of a coronary artery limits the increase to the blood flow and pain arises from the oxygen-deprived (ischaemic) heart muscle.

This sequence of events is called 'stable' angina, but sometimes anginal pain becomes more prolonged or occurs when the person is not exercising. It is then called 'unstable' angina and, because it can be followed by a heart attack, it needs prompt treatment. Such treatment is very effective if given early.

Major rhythm abnormality

The most serious form of coronary heart disease is a dramatic collapse due to sudden failure of the pumping action. This failure is caused by a major abnormality in the rhythm of the heart beat, most often a disorder called ventricular fibrillation.

When this happens, there is a rapid loss of consciousness, sometimes preceded by chest pain, and the sufferer may die within

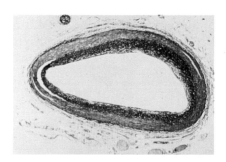

Cross-section of a normal aorta (main artery).

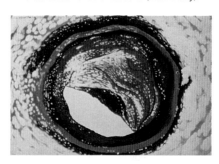

Aorta narrowed by atherosclerotic plaques.

minutes unless prompt, effective resuscitation is given and he is taken to hospital.

One common culprit

All these forms of coronary heart disease result from narrowing of the coronary arteries, which reduces the flow of oxygen-bearing blood to the muscular walls of the heart. So we shall now look more closely at this disease process.

ATHEROSCLEROSIS

The main disease process that thickens and distorts the inner lining of all arteries is called atherosclerosis. In countries in which heart attack is common (such as Britain and the USA), early signs of atherosclerosis can be seen in childhood. The damage does not develop in the whole blood vessel – it is patchy. The affected areas of the artery lining are known as atherosclerotic plaques and these enlarge progressively and can bulge into the cavity of the artery. This process need not narrow the artery to a serious extent until other changes begin to happen. However, further changes can be rapid, and when they occur they may convert a symptomless, slowly developing disorder into one of the dramatic forms of heart disease already described. Let us look at what happens step by step.

How does it begin?

Atherosclerosis begins when certain white blood cells stick to the lining of the artery. Soon they get through the lining and come to lie just beneath the surface of the artery wall. They then begin to collect droplets of fatty substances, particularly cholesterol, and this gives the cells a foamy appearance. The cholesterol in the cells of the plaques comes from the cholesterol in the blood, particularly in the form of tiny particles called low density lipoprotein or LDL (see *Understanding lipids* on page 23). A high blood cholesterol level is most often due to an excess of LDL in the blood, as these particles are rich in cholesterol. The higher the level of LDL in the blood, the more rapidly cholesterol accumulates in the wall of the artery, and the faster the plaques grow in size.

A heart attack in a man of 50 years of age has its origins in the process of atherosclerosis that began 30 or more years earlier

A further reason for the thickening of the arterial wall is that large numbers of muscle cells collect in the inner lining. These cells also secrete a fibrous material called collagen.

Segment of artery wall

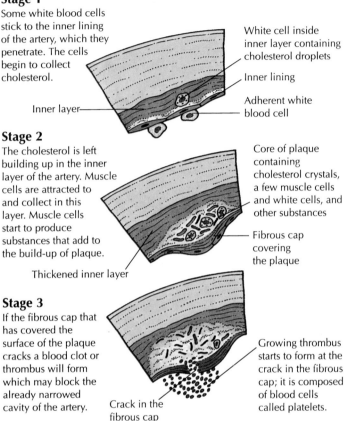

Stage 1
Some white blood cells stick to the inner lining of the artery, which they penetrate. The cells begin to collect cholesterol.

White cell inside inner layer containing cholesterol droplets

Inner lining

Inner layer

Adherent white blood cell

Stage 2
The cholesterol is left building up in the inner layer of the artery. Muscle cells are attracted to and collect in this layer. Muscle cells start to produce substances that add to the build-up of plaque.

Core of plaque containing cholesterol crystals, a few muscle cells and white cells, and other substances

Fibrous cap covering the plaque

Thickened inner layer

Stage 3
If the fibrous cap that has covered the surface of the plaque cracks a blood clot or thrombus will form which may block the already narrowed cavity of the artery.

Crack in the fibrous cap

Growing thrombus starts to form at the crack in the fibrous cap; it is composed of blood cells called platelets.

Stages in the formation of an atheromatous plaque.

When the surface splits
The additional, sometimes catastrophic changes that lead to a heart attack start with the splitting open of the fibrous coat over the surface of the plaque in one of the coronary arteries. When this happens, tiny blood cells called platelets stick to the newly exposed interior of the plaque and the rapid build-up of layer upon layer of these platelets forms a blood clot (called a thrombus).

This can rapidly block or further reduce the cavity of the already narrowed artery and deprive part of the heart muscle of its blood supply; as described earlier, this can cause a heart attack, unstable angina or ventricular fibrillation. This damaging sequence of events is most likely to happen to quite small plaques in which large quantities of cholesterol have collected.

The secondary process of thrombosis (clotting) rapidly changes this atherosclerotic narrowing into the more complete blockage which then causes a heart attack.

It's a long process

These changes develop slowly over many years. A heart attack in a man of 50 years of age has its origins in the process of atherosclerosis that began 30 or more years earlier.

Coronary spasm

Other events play an important part in the narrowing of the coronary arteries. When the muscle in deeper layers of the artery wall contracts (called a coronary spasm), the moderate narrowing due to the atherosclerosis may become severe enough to restrict blood flow. This often happens near an atherosclerotic plaque and can lead to a serious but reversible lack of blood supply to the heart muscle. The result is often an episode of angina, with the patient feeling pain in the chest.

The smooth cells which line the arteries normally produce a substance that relaxes the muscle in the artery wall and so enhances the blood flow through them. When the blood cholesterol level is high, this process becomes faulty; and it can fail completely when arteries develop atherosclerosis. As a result, less blood will flow through the coronary arteries to the heart muscle.

Laboratory experiments have shown that lowering a high level of blood cholesterol can rapidly restore the relaxing mechanism and improve blood flow.

Is atherosclerosis inevitable?

The sequence of events does not happen, or happens to only a minor extent, in people who have only low levels of cholesterol in their blood. So the amount of cholesterol in the blood plays a central role in the processes of atherosclerosis.

We discuss what cholesterol is, what controls it and how it can harm the arteries on page 23, *Understanding lipids.*

Causes of heart attack

In this chapter, we discuss the several known causes of coronary disease – for heart attack is no longer a mystery. We don't yet have all the answers, but we have a good understanding of its major causes, and as individuals we can do a lot to reduce our chances of having a heart attack.

In Australia and the USA, for example, where experts were quick off the mark in the 1960s in telling the public about this new knowledge, deaths from coronary disease have halved in the last 20 years. American figures for 1988/90 show deaths from heart disease decreased by 6.3 per cent, and the total death rate decreased by 2.3 per cent, within a single year.

BLOOD CHOLESTEROL AND DIET

The greater the amount of cholesterol in the blood, the higher the risk of having a heart attack. The risk is about four times higher in a man whose cholesterol is around 7.5 mmol/l (cholesterol is measured in millimoles per litre of blood plasma) than in one whose level is around 5 mmol/l. Risk increases even more steeply in people whose cholesterol level is still higher. Those who have the inherited disease called familial hypercholesterolaemia have levels of 8 to 14 mmol/l, and men affected by this disorder have at least a ten times greater risk of coronary heart disease than men with average cholesterol levels (around 6 mmol/l).

Although we know less about very low levels of cholesterol, cholesterol levels below 5 mmol/l are accompanied by even less risk, although the difference is not so great. In this sense, the lower the cholesterol the better; there are very low levels in rural parts of China (around 3 mmol/l), where coronary disease is extremely rare. The target for most of us is a cholesterol level near 5 mmol/l. It is not easy to get the level much below this, and the decrease in risk is proportionally smaller. Today 5.2 mmol/l is regarded as the desirable upper limit for most adults. While this figure is a useful guide, doctors interpret it quite flexibly because someone's risk of having a heart attack depends on many factors in addition to cholesterol level. So a somewhat higher cholesterol level is acceptable if there are no other risk factors whereas in someone whose overall risk of heart disease is high, the doctor may set the target level of blood cholesterol even lower than 5.2 mmol/l (see *High cholesterol – lowering the risk*, on page 38).

National comparisons

When we compare different countries we find wide variation between them in average cholesterol levels, and the death rates from heart attack vary in proportion to the average blood cholesterol level. In Scotland and Northern Ireland, deaths from heart attack are about ten times more common than in Japan, for example. The main reason for the differences in average blood cholesterol is the

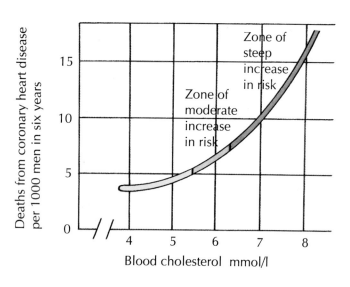

The further the cholesterol is lowered, the greater the reduction in coronary disease.

contrasting food habits in the various countries. In particular, the amount of animal fat eaten in the diet is much lower in countries with low average cholesterol levels and low rates of heart attack. There seems to be no disadvantage in having the very low cholesterol levels seen in these countries. Men and women in Japan live longer than people in Scotland and in most other countries in Northern Europe where fat intake and average blood cholesterol are higher.

BENEFITS OF LOWERING CHOLESTEROL

Lessens heart attack risks

Powerful evidence for this statement comes from the results of some 30 controlled clinical trials. In such trials, one group of people receive a treatment to lower their blood cholesterol (diet, a drug or an operation), while a closely similar group do not receive such treatment. The numbers of events such as heart attacks in the two groups are compared after a period of between two and ten years.

When most of the trials are considered separately, and when the results are pooled to give information on around 40,000 participants, the evidence shows that reducing blood cholesterol lessens the chance of heart attack. The further the cholesterol level is lowered, the greater the reduction in coronary disease. Although atherosclerosis may take decades to develop, lowering cholesterol for only three to five years removes most of the risk caused by having high blood cholesterol.

For example, in one recent trial of a widely used cholesterol-lowering drug in people who already had coronary disease, fatal heart attacks were reduced by 42 per cent, all heart attacks by 34 per cent, and the need for operations by 37 per cent. In fact the chance of dying from any cause decreased by 30 per cent. Benefit was seen in both men and women, and in middle-aged as well as elderly people.

Can widen narrowed coronary arteries

This conclusion is based on a further 16 controlled trials of lowering cholesterol, plus a number of less rigorous studies. X-rays of the coronary arteries were taken just before treatment began, and again between one and ten years later. Changes between the first and second X-ray were assessed by a panel of heart specialists or by a computerized device that measured the width of the artery with amazing accuracy.

The results were highly consistent. In groups not receiving any cholesterol-lowering treatment, coronary arteries and their branches tended to become narrower, and spontaneous improvement was very rare. In the groups receiving treatment, the tendency towards any further narrowing was significantly lessened, and improvement was seen much more commonly. In some of the trials, patients who were treated to reduce cholesterol suffered fewer heart attacks, which is clear evidence of the medical value of the treatment. Two trials were large enough, and long enough, to show that when the coronary arteries improved in the first three years of the study, the risk of heart attack was reduced in the fourth to tenth years.

The same happens in laboratory animals

The link between cholesterol and atherosclerosis was established more than 80 years ago when some army doctors in St Petersburg fed their pet rabbit with high-cholesterol scraps from the mess table – with fatal results. The arteries of laboratory animals develop atherosclerosis when the normally low blood cholesterol levels become raised. This happens in strains of rabbits in which a high blood cholesterol is inherited and in several species of animal when fed a diet that increases blood cholesterol levels.

Atherosclerosis in such animals shows a considerable degree of healing when the blood cholesterol is lowered by diet or by a drug. Much of the cholesterol disappears from the plaques in the walls of the arteries, and the ability of the arteries to relax is restored. Both effects lead to a wider artery. In animals with inherited high cholesterol levels, giving a cholesterol-lowering drug early in life almost completely prevents atherosclerosis.

What brings about the benefit?

Lowering raised blood cholesterol levels slows progressive growth of atherosclerotic plaques in coronary arteries and, just as with animals, even causes shrinkage of these plaques. This gives benefit simply because it allows improved blood flow to the heart muscle, but other effects may be even more valuable. As we have seen, plaques, and high blood cholesterol itself, prevent the normal process that keeps the muscle in the walls of the arteries relaxed (see page 4). As a result the muscle contracts and so narrows the arteries. The relaxation process is restored when the blood cholesterol level is lowered, and so the blood flow through the coronary arteries is improved.

Perhaps the most important benefit is that there is less chance that the plaque will split open and completely close a blood vessel with a clot (thrombus – see page 7). Such splitting is most likely to happen to plaques that contain a lot of cholesterol covered by only a thin layer of fibrous coat. It may be that lowering the blood cholesterol decreases the amount of cholesterol in these plaques and lessens the number of damaging foamy white cells (described on page 7) sufficiently to stabilize them and to avoid the risk of splitting and clot formation.

Who benefits?

The evidence from all the research done so far clearly shows that benefits of cholesterol lowering are seen:

- in men and in women
- in previously healthy people
- in those who have already had a heart attack
- in the middle-aged and (in the one trial on older people) in the over-sixties.

The benefits are seen in parts of coronary arteries that were severely narrowed by atherosclerosis and also in moderately affected or near-normal parts.

Whatever the treatment, the benefit is noticeable even within one to two years.

What can be done?

We are still not sure about all the details, but there is enough information now for all of us to make practical decisions about diet and blood cholesterol which will lessen our chances of having a heart attack. We know that the risk is highest in people with the highest cholesterol levels, and we know that this risk is reduced by lowering the cholesterol level. The more the cholesterol is lowered, the bigger the fall in the risk of heart attack.

Cholesterol is not the only risk factor for a heart attack. Before we go on to look at cholesterol in more detail – what it is and how it affects us – we shall finish this chapter by dealing with the other risk factors which also increase the risk of heart attack.

OTHER RISK FACTORS

Smoking and heart attack

Cigarette smoking increases the chance of having a heart attack. It also encourages atherosclerosis in the legs and other parts of the body, which can lead to other serious medical conditions. The more you smoke, the greater the risk. Studies on people who have quit the habit show that the risk of having a heart attack decreases steeply, and quite soon after they stop. For smokers who have already had a heart attack, giving up cigarettes will halve the chance of a second attack.

Effects of smoking

We do not fully understand how smoking leads to these harmful effects but we know that:

- smoking increases the conversion of LDL to a modified chemical product which has a special ability to carry cholesterol into the cells of the walls of arteries (see *Understanding lipids* on pages 7 and 22);
- smoking increases the tendency of blood platelets to stick together, leading to formation of a blood clot (thrombus);
- smoking also lowers the level of high density lipoprotein (HDL) in the blood, lessening the protection apparently provided by this substance (see page 29).

High blood pressure

High blood pressure is another important risk factor for heart attack. The higher the blood pressure, the greater the chance of having coronary disease. Even mildly raised blood pressure means a measurable increase in risk. So it is important to have your blood pressure checked regularly.

We know from many clinical trials that lowering high blood pressure greatly reduces the risk of having a stroke, and heart failure due to high blood pressure can largely be avoided. More recent trials (and the pooled results of the many earlier ones) also show a reduction in the risk of heart attack; these benefits are seen after age 60 (when high blood pressure is very common) as well as in middle age. High blood pressure is reduced by losing surplus weight, by cutting down the intake of alcohol and of salt and, when necessary, by various drugs which can be highly effective.

Diabetes

If you have diabetes, you are at increased risk of heart attack and of atherosclerosis affecting the legs. We know that all the other risk factors, like high blood pressure, high blood cholesterol and smoking, are even more harmful when diabetes is also present. So avoiding these risk factors is particularly important if you have diabetes. Diabetes also tends to raise the levels of triglyceride (fat) and other lipids in blood, some of which is carried in the small lipoprotein particles that seem to be particularly damaging to the artery (see page 29).

The more cholesterol is lowered, the bigger the fall in the risk of heart attack

Today, the diet that is prescribed to help diabetes is designed not only to control the high blood sugar and to achieve a correct body

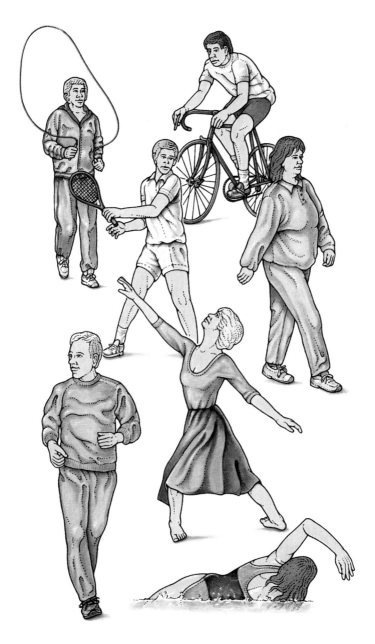

The most valuable kind of exercise is called aerobic.

weight, but also to reduce the levels of cholesterol and fat (triglyceride) in the blood.

Additional risks

There are several other coronary risk factors for which the scientific evidence is persuasive, although the evidence is less complete than for the three factors we have already discussed.

Obesity

As we shall see (page 21), people who are overweight, especially those who carry their extra pounds around their abdomen, have an increased risk of heart attack.

Obesity increases the likelihood that someone will have other known risk factors for heart disease; these include high blood pressure, diabetes, high blood cholesterol and triglyceride levels, and deficiency of the protective HDL. In addition, obesity round the trunk directly increases the risk of heart attack and worsens angina. There are many other ill effects of obesity and there is every reason (including stamina and self-esteem) to shed any surplus weight.

Losing weight is one of the most effective treatments for moderately high blood cholesterol and triglyceride, moderately high blood pressure and for the common form of diabetes.

Heavy drinking

Heavy drinkers have a greatly increased risk of heart attack and stroke, partly because they tend to have high blood pressure and are often overweight.

Lack of regular exercise

Regular exercise is part of a healthy way of life, and many research findings suggest that it may help protect against heart attack. Exercise helps combat obesity, reduces the blood fat (triglyceride) level and lowers the blood glucose level in diabetics.

The most valuable kind of exercise is called aerobic. This is the type that it makes you breathe more deeply and increases your pulse rate, for example brisk walking, jogging, swimming, cycling and games like tennis.

One of the benefits is a progressive increase in the amount of protective HDL in the blood. Furthermore, people who exercise regularly seem to be able to clear cholesterol from their blood stream more easily than those who do not.

If you are not used to exercising and are middle-aged or older, you should ask your doctor's advice before undertaking an exercise programme.

You should also do so if you think you are at high risk of heart disease. Exercise should leave you pleasantly tired, and you should be fully recovered within five minutes. You should start gently and increase gradually over several months, working up to about three hours per week, exercising daily or on alternate days.

Stress

Certain stresses are an added risk factor in people who are at risk of heart attack from other causes, notably an unbalanced diet and a high blood cholesterol level,

You cannot avoid stress completely, but it is particularly important for those who are often in a stressful situation to deal effectively with all the other risk factors. The worst answer to stress is to reach for another cigarette or a drink.

Many people still believe that the overworked executive is at high risk of a heart attack. But deaths from coronary heart disease are more common in manual workers than in businessmen. This is because the really important risks are bad diet, smoking and high blood pressure, and nowadays the more privileged person, the businessman and his friends, are more likely to have heeded medical advice on healthy living. Unfortunately the less privileged have not improved their health habits to the same extent.

Other factors

Recent research has been shown that heart attack risk is also affected by the amount of other substances in the blood. Doctors are increasingly aware of the risks caused by excess fibrinogen and lipoprotein (a), for example.

Understanding lipids

In order to understand what cholesterol is, how it gets into the lining of the artery and what controls our cholesterol levels, we will take a closer look at it and other fat-like substances in the body.

Cholesterol

Cholesterol is the best known of a group of fat-like substances in the body called lipids. A certain amount of cholesterol is essential to life, and it is present in every cell in the body and also in blood plasma.

Cholesterol has three distinct roles in the body:

- it is a necessary part of the membranes that surround the body's cells;
- it is needed by the liver to make bile, which helps to digest our food;
- it is used by hormone-producing glands to make certain hormones – the body's chemical messengers.

Lipoproteins

Because cholesterol and all the other lipids are not soluble in water, the body has evolved a special way of carrying them around in the blood stream. It does this by building them into particles called lipoproteins, which are soluble in water and in blood plasma.

Each particle of lipoprotein contains cholesterol and other lipids (including ordinary fat, called triglyceride) attached to special protein carriers called apoproteins. There are various types of lipoproteins, each with different proportions of these substances. They are mainly classified by how dense (heavy) they are, such as low density lipoprotein, and each type of lipoprotein has a different function.

How does cholesterol get into the arteries?

As we have seen, cholesterol is carried in blood plasma in

lipoproteins. About two-thirds of the cholesterol in the blood is in low density lipoprotein (LDL for short), and if you have high levels of cholesterol in the blood this is usually because you have too much LDL. The LDL filters from blood plasma into the wall of the artery and the higher the level of the LDL (or cholesterol) in your blood the more it filters into the arterial wall and accumulates there.

Before LDL can enter the cells of the artery wall in significant amounts, it undergoes a chemical change. This modified LDL is rapidly taken up by certain white blood cells in the artery wall, and cholesterol accumulates in and thickens the wall as these cells die. One such chemical change, studied a lot recently, results from the action of oxygen on the LDL – a process known as LDL oxidation. This may be a very important step in the development of atherosclerosis and coronary disease. If so, prevention of LDL oxidation could reduce coronary disease. Studies on laboratory animals suggest that this is so, but we must await clinical trials to be sure.

Meanwhile it is reassuring that the diet described on pages 46–9 for treating a high cholesterol level is a good source of the anti-oxidant vitamins (vitamin C, beta-carotene and vitamin E) that can reduce the damaging LDL oxidation in your body.

A high blood cholesterol level is one of the most potent causes of coronary heart disease

Other effects of a high cholesterol level

We know that the earliest stage of atherosclerosis – when certain white blood cells stick to and enter the lining of the arterial wall – is also stimulated by high levels of blood cholesterol.

We know, too, that the formation of a thrombus, or clot – the serious complication that can block a coronary artery – is more likely to happen when cholesterol levels are high, apparently because a lot of LDL in the blood can alter the 'stickiness' of blood platelets, encouraging clot formation.

The link between cholesterol and coronaries

These processes explain why people with high levels of LDL in the blood (and therefore high levels of cholesterol) have a high risk of suffering from heart attack. There is no longer any serious dispute about this: a high blood cholesterol level is one of the most potent causes of coronary heart disease.

We next need to understand why so many people have undesirably high blood cholesterol levels.

What controls blood cholesterol levels?

The short answers to this very important question are:

- Our diet
- Our genes.

Other factors certainly contribute – hormones, exercise and commonly used drugs such as diuretics and anti-acne drugs – but in this chapter we concentrate on the two main influences.

CALORIES AND CORONARIES

We have already mentioned the dangers of obesity, but the message is important enough to be worth re-stating. The amount we eat (and drink) influences our weight, which in turn affects our risk of having a coronary, as well as many other diseases. The amount of energy we spend, at rest and during physical activity, varies enormously among different people. Obesity can run in families because the difference in resting energy expenditure can have a genetic basis. But whatever its basis, it is unfortunately true that being overweight increases the chance of having a heart attack.

Why obesity increases the chances of heart disease

The reasons for this are numerous. Overweight people tend to have higher levels of cholesterol and fat in their blood plasma, and they usually have lower levels of cholesterol in their HDL, some of which may help protect against heart attack as they mop up surplus cholesterol from the cells. They also tend to have higher blood pressure

and to be at greater risk of developing diabetes.

The danger of middle-aged spread

It seems that putting on weight in early middle-age is particularly risky. Those of us who fail to keep the slender figures of our early 20s, allowing our weight to creep up in adult life, have higher cholesterol levels and higher blood pressure than those whose self discipline is sterner and whose genes are kinder. It also appears that the risk of heart disease depends on where we store our extra pounds. Excess fat in the abdominal region – common in men – is more hazardous than extra inches on the hips and thighs.

Benefits of weight reduction

Getting rid of those surplus pounds is beneficial. In people who are even moderately overweight, a period of weight reduction substantially lowers their blood cholesterol and fat levels, improves HDL levels, lessens blood pressure and helps control diabetes.

OUR EATING HABITS

Food is not our only source of cholesterol – about half of our body's cholesterol is manufactured by the liver and other tissues. So we do not need to eat any cholesterol in our food. Increasing the amount of cholesterol we eat increases blood cholesterol levels in most people. In a few, this is a powerful effect, but in others it is negligible. This is because we vary in the extent to which our blood cholesterol level increases when we eat foods containing cholesterol and/or fat.

If you change your diet so that you replace saturated fats with unsaturated fats and oils, your blood cholesterol falls

Egg yolks, kidneys and other offal, shellfish such as shrimps and prawns and, to a small extent, all animal products, are high in cholesterol.

Turning to the individual components of our diet, we will concentrate on fats as they are so important in determining how much cholesterol we have in our blood. Fibre also plays a useful part in lowering cholesterol.

FATS

There are two main types of fat: saturated and unsaturated. These terms refer to their different chemical natures but they also look different and have very different effects on our body.

Saturated fats

This is the chemical term for those fats that tend to be hard at room temperature, like most meat fats and butter (animal fats) and hard margarines and cooking fats (which are processed vegetable fats).

These fats (the triglycerides) are chemical compounds of glycerol and substances called fatty acids, each of which have long chains of carbon atoms. Most common among the fatty acids which make up saturated fats are those with 16, 14 or 12 carbon atoms, and foods containing these are – unfortunately – very effective in increasing our blood cholesterol and the level of LDL in our blood.

Effects of saturated fat

The more we eat these foods, the higher our blood cholesterol level, and the higher the risk of heart attack. When we eat less saturated fat, however, our blood cholesterol level falls promptly (within three weeks). Because of this, the main principle behind a diet for reducing the risk of coronary disease is to limit foods rich in saturated fat to, at most, one-half of the typical British intake. This would mean reducing the amount of calories we obtain from saturated fats to less than 10 per cent of our total calorie intake.

Examples of foods high in saturated fat are:

- fatty kinds of meat
- cream
- butter
- whole-fat milk and cheeses
- baked foods like biscuits and cakes that are made with saturated shortenings
- hard margarines
- coconut
- chocolate.

Fortunately, there is a wide range of enjoyable foods to replace those that should be avoided. Also, we vary widely in the extent to which our blood cholesterol is affected by saturated fats.

Unsaturated fats

Unsaturated fats are liquid or soft solids at room temperature, and

chemically are chiefly made up of unsaturated fatty acids. Chemists among us may know that unsaturated carbon chains are kinked at points where the carbon atoms are joined by 'double bonds', and these kinks result in the soft or liquid consistency. It is enough to know that sunflower oil, corn oil or olive oil and certain soft margarines are examples of unsaturated fats. When the fatty acid has one double bond it is called monounsaturated, and when it has two or more it is polyunsaturated. A common monounsaturated fat is olive oil, whereas sunflower oil and margarine made from it are polyunsaturated.

Effects of unsaturated fats

If you change your diet so that you replace saturated fats with

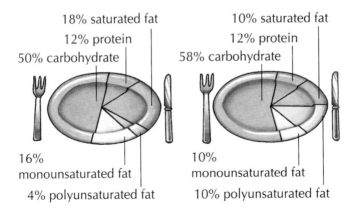

18% saturated fat
12% protein
50% carbohydrate
16% monounsaturated fat
4% polyunsaturated fat

10% saturated fat
12% protein
58% carbohydrate
10% monounsaturated fat
10% polyunsaturated fat

A diet rich in saturated fat (left) and a cholesterol-lowering diet (right).

unsaturated fats and oils, your blood cholesterol decreases. This is partly the result of eating less saturated fat, but adding polyunsaturated fat lowers the cholesterol further.

This can be shown by measuring the reduction in the cholesterol level when saturated fat in the diet is replaced by starchy foods, for example carbohydrate. The blood cholesterol falls substantially, but the fall is not as great as when polyunsaturated fat, rather than carbohydrate, replaces the saturated fat.

Many experts believe that the major type of polyunsaturated fat, in which linoleic acid is the main fatty acid and which is found largely in seed oils such as sunflower oil, should provide 6 to 8 per cent of our food energy. At present it varies from 2.5 to 6.0 per cent in different countries.

What about monounsaturated fat?

Like polyunsaturated fat, replacement of saturated fat in the diet by monounsaturated fat leads to a fall

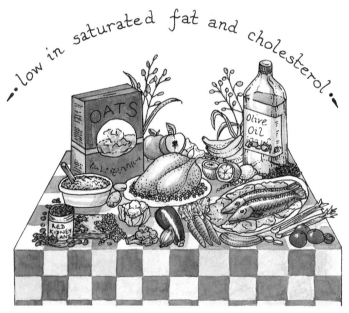

low in saturated fat and cholesterol

olive oil · vegetables · pulses · oats · citrus fruit berries, apples & bananas · fish, chicken & lean meat

in blood cholesterol level. It is therefore reasonable to use an oil such as olive oil in your diet; it contains mainly monounsaturated fatty acids.

The ideal balance of mono-unsaturated and polyunsaturated fats in your diet has not yet been worked out.

Fat intake

Until we know more, it seems best to keep our intake of all kinds of fat quite low. This is especially true of saturated fat, but we should use no more than moderate amounts of both types of unsaturated fat. Clearly a little unsaturated oil in a dressing makes a salad more palatable, as does a fat-reduced polyunsaturated margarine used as a spread. But we should remember that all kinds of fat are calorie-rich. The diet in the parts of the world in which heart attack is rarest is usually very low in fat and high in carbohydrate.

There seem to be no magical health-giving properties in a diet rich in unsaturated fats.

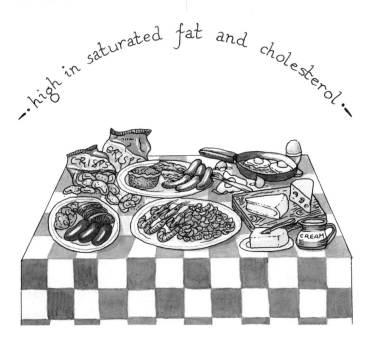

...high in saturated fat and cholesterol...

kidneys & offal • cream, butter, full fat cheese
egg yolks • crisps • fatty meat products • shrimps & prawns

Other benefits of polyunsaturated fats

Polyunsaturated fats benefit the body in other ways. Their effect on blood clotting (thrombosis) is opposite to that of saturated fats. Increased intake of polyunsaturates reduces the tendency to form clots (thrombi). It has also been repeatedly found that heart attacks happen less often in people who have a high proportion of linoleic acid (a polyunsaturated fatty acid) in their tissues than in those with less of this acid.

Triglyceride, HDL and coronaries

Although we do not know for certain whether high triglyceride (fat) levels in the blood are a cause of heart attack, there are increasing grounds for believing this to be so. We know that LDL circulating in the blood causes atherosclerosis. In people with high levels of triglyceride in their blood, the LDL particles are smaller than in other people, and it seems that small LDL particles are particularly likely to cause atherosclerosis.

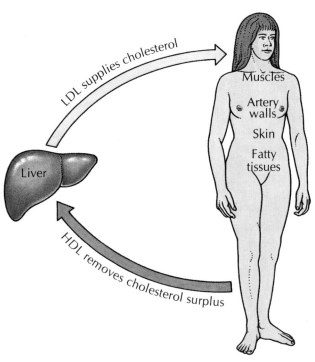

Transport of cholesterol in LDL and HDL.

One difficulty is that a high triglyceride level rarely occurs alone. It is usually found with other risk factors for coronary heart disease, such as obesity, lack of HDL and diabetes. People who drink too much alcohol also tend to have high triglyceride levels.

● **Lowering triglyceride levels:** the blood triglyceride level is lowered by correcting obesity, by eating unsaturated fats of all kinds, especially those found in fatty fish such as mackerel and herring, by exercise, and by cutting down on alcohol.

● **The lipoprotein transport network:** lipoproteins in the blood are rather like traffic in a two-lane road – they carry cholesterol in both directions. Lipoproteins such as LDL carry lipids outwards, from the liver and gut to other parts of the body such as muscles, skin, fatty tissue and also artery walls. Cholesterol is carried outwards chiefly in LDL. But to maintain the balance there has to be a two-way traffic, with a comparable amount of cholesterol leaving these tissues. This reverse traffic in cholesterol is initially carried in HDL, one type of which helps to pick up surplus cholesterol from the cells.

● **Low HDL increases risk of a coronary:** people with low levels of HDL cholesterol (for example less than 0.9 mmol/l) in their blood plasma have a greater risk of developing coronary disease. This is probably because they are less able than others to clear cholesterol from the walls of the arteries.

● **Low HDL levels are common in obese people and in smokers:** thin people who take regular exercise have higher levels and women have more HDL in blood than men. Undesirably low levels can run in families.

The benefits of fibre

There are many kinds of dietary fibre, but one group, often called soluble fibre, is effective in lowering blood cholesterol level if you eat enough of it. Unprocessed foods of plant origin such as vegetables, pulses (such as dried beans and lentils), fruit (especially berries, bananas, apples and citrus fruits) and some cereals (oats but not wheat) are good sources of soluble fibre.

Remember that all of these dietary effects add up. So, making several modest changes to your diet will often have a large effect on blood cholesterol.

EFFECT OF INHERITANCE

We all know that heart attacks sometimes run in families. When experts in genetics have measured the importance of inheritance, however, they have come up with a variety of answers. A commonly held view is that one-third of the difference in risk between people may be inherited, whereas two-thirds result from our environment and, in particular, our own behaviour (for example, eating an unbalanced diet, smoking or not taking enough exercise). We have already seen that heart attacks are comparatively rare in countries where the diet is low in fat, such as Japan. However, when Japanese people emigrate to Hawaii and California, they rapidly become prone to heart attack, showing that their former protection was chiefly due to the Japanese way of life rather than being inherited.

• **Inherited susceptibility:** all the same, differences in blood cholesterol levels and in heart attack rates between countries may, in small part, be due to genetic differences. When we look at the differences in blood cholesterol levels within one country, genes play a much bigger role as within one country people do not differ widely in dietary habits. Recent research suggests that we may inherit a differing susceptibility to the cholesterol-raising effect of the fat and cholesterol in our diet. This is not all bad news: people who have a high blood cholesterol level because of an inherited suscept-ibility will also tend to show a large fall in the blood cholesterol level when they reduce the amount of fat they eat. Such differences between

people probably reflect the combined effect of not just one but several genes.

• **Other risk factors may be inherited too:** family proneness to coronary disease can also reflect the fact that other risk factors, notably diabetes, high blood pressure and obesity are also, in part, inherited diseases. The level of another risk

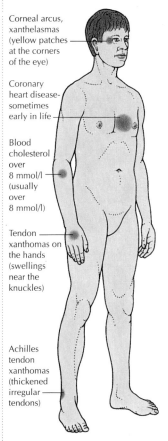

Corneal arcus, xanthelasmas (yellow patches at the corners of the eye)

Coronary heart disease-sometimes early in life

Blood cholesterol over 8 mmol/l (usually over 8 mmol/l)

Tendon xanthomas on the hands (swellings near the knuckles)

Achilles tendon xanthomas (thickened irregular tendons)

Signs of inherited high cholesterol levels.

factor, lipoprotein (a), in the blood is also influenced by our genes.

Inherited conditions that affect cholesterol levels

There are a few conditions in which the blood cholesterol, and sometimes the blood triglyceride (fat) levels are high, even very high, as a result of inheriting a single gene. These disorders often run strongly in families, although they may not know it: this is strong justification for widespread testing of healthy people for high blood cholesterol.

• **Familial hypercholesterolaemia:** we have already mentioned one of these conditions, familial hyper-cholesterolaemia. In its relatively common form, there are about 120,000 affected people in Britain,

and they are at high risk of coronary disease. This can occur in the 40s, 30s or even the 20s in men and somewhat later in women. Their blood cholesterol level is high from birth, and by adulthood is usually very high (8 to 14 mmol/l whereas it averages about 5.7 mmol/l in normal British people). The condition is strongly inherited: one parent is always affected and about half of each generation carries the gene. Several members of the family may therefore be afflicted by heart trouble at an early age. Treatment requires diet and a drug in order to lower the very high cholesterol level sufficiently. By taking repeated X-rays of the coronary arteries it has been shown that when blood cholesterol is effectively lowered in those with

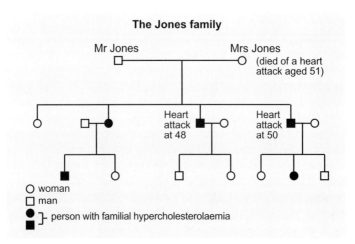

The Jones family

Family tree showing the inheritance of hypercholesterolaemia and the occurrence of heart attack.

this condition, previously narrowed arteries can become wider again.

• **Remnant hyperlipidaemia:** somewhat less common is a disorder called remnant hyperlipidaemia. In people with this disorder, both the cholesterol and triglyceride levels are usually very high, with the result that the coronary arteries, the arteries to the legs and sometimes also those to the brain become narrowed. This condition responds particularly well to diet and drug treatment.

• **Other inherited conditions:** lead to a rather milder increase in blood cholesterol levels and treatment by diet returns the levels to normal in most affected people. These disorders are far commoner than the severer ones just described.

Have you inherited a high cholesterol level?

• **Xanthomas:** sometimes your doctor can recognize tell-tale deposits of cholesterol in the skin or tendons, known as xanthomas. In familial hypercholesterolaemia, these may look like split-pea-shaped swellings in the tendons near the knuckles, or sometimes they are large irregular lumps behind the ankles. In remnant hyperlipidaemia these may be roundish, pink or orange swellings, most often over the elbows, and orange lines in the creases of the palms. It must be stressed,

however, that many people with these disorders do not have xanthomas and the only way to be sure of the diagnosis is to take a blood sample and measure the cholesterol and triglyceride levels and sometimes the lipoprotein values.

• **Other physical signs:** other outward signs are less reliable. They may lead to a suspicion that the cholesterol level is high, but are far

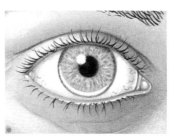

Cornea shows a white crescent (corneal arcus).

from specific. One (called an arcus) takes the form of a white ring or crescent in the outer part of the cornea of the eye, where it shows up against the brown or blue colour. People with this sign who are under age 30 usually have raised cholesterol and in those up to age 60 this is quite often the case; but the sign is not a good indicator beyond the age of 60.

Another comparable sign takes the form of yellow, flattish spots – xanthelasmas – on the eyelids. Again, when this is seen in young people it often indicates high cholesterol, but it is also quite common with normal levels of cholesterol.

• **More subtle genetic effects:** we have recently learned about other, more subtle ways in which genes can lead to high cholesterol levels or cause a high risk of heart attack without a particularly high blood cholesterol level. For example, we inherit higher or lower levels of the apoprotein called apo (a), which is carried in LDL. This possibly affects blood clotting processes, and having a high level gives a somewhat increased risk of a heart attack.

Much research is going on in this area, although it has not led to new ways of reducing heart disease.

High cholesterol – lowering the risk

Let us start by listing three facts that have been discussed in earlier parts of this book:

- high cholesterol levels are a cause of heart attack;
- we know with certainty that reducing high cholesterol levels lessens the risk of heart attack;
- the only way to know if the level of cholesterol is high is to measure it in a blood sample.

As heart attacks and coronary heart disease in general are exceedingly common in Britain, it is essential that we deal with the problem. The most important way is to prevent it happening in the first place. Prevention depends on reducing all risk factors that can be altered. Of these, high cholesterol levels have, until recently, received less attention than they should. Most experts have concluded that blood cholesterol levels should be measured in all adults as one of the necessary steps in reducing coronary disease. I strongly support this view, and will return to it shortly.

The other way is to treat those who have coronary disease to reduce the risk of further attacks.

Prevention – the healthy living approach

We can all reduce our cholesterol levels to some extent by adopting a healthier way of life, by eating the kind of diet outlined on page 46 and by avoiding obesity. This would shift the present range of blood cholesterol levels in the whole population downwards, to a lower and safer national range.

This approach, which depends on educating all of us about healthier living, is essential if we are to reduce the toll taken by heart attacks.

It's not enough

But unfortunately this means of reducing cholesterol levels is not enough on its own. This is partly because it is a slow process, and reaches different groups in the population very unevenly. There is also another weakness in this approach. Many people with high levels of blood cholesterol find that they cannot lower it sufficiently by diet alone. Some serious conditions do respond to diet, but many people with relatively high levels need to diet under the supervision of a doctor or dietician if they are to achieve a safe level of cholesterol; and many of those with high levels may need a drug as well as the diet. They need the second strategy – the medical approach.

MEDICAL APPROACH

This approach requires that high cholesterol levels, like high blood pressure, should be diagnosed by a doctor and treated under supervision. If your cholesterol is high (more than 6.5 mmol/l) you will be given a diet and the improvement will be checked after a few months by a further blood test. If necessary, the doctor, nurse or dietician will give further guidance about the diet, together with the encouragement that is part of medical care. It may take a year to maximize the benefit that the new eating habits can provide. For patients with very high levels (as in familial hypercholesterolaemia) and for the few with relatively high levels that are not reduced by careful dieting, the doctor may advise drug treatment in addition to diet, or may refer such people to a hospital lipid clinic.

A health check is necessary

If this medical approach is to be used at all, it depends on carrying out cholesterol tests on all adults who are likely to benefit – and also on children who have a parent with a disease such as familial hypercholesterolaemia, or a close relative who has developed coronary disease at an early age (see *How much treatment is needed* on page 43).

There are several benefits to including cholesterol measurement in the health check:

- diagnosing the serious inherited conditions that cause a high cholesterol level and lead to a very high risk of coronary disease if not treated;
- recognizing the less severe but commoner high cholesterol levels that respond best to supervised care by a doctor;
- providing motivation to follow the healthy living approach – if we know that our cholesterol is higher than it should be, we will know how important these

changes in living habits are to us personally.

How is the blood test done?

There is no single best way of testing people. Some general practices run schemes in which they offer you an appointment to have a health check. When you attend, you will be seen by the practice nurse or the doctor. You will be asked about your family background – in particular whether any close relatives had heart troubles, and you will be asked if you smoke. Your weight, height and blood pressure will be recorded. Finally, a small blood sample will be taken from a vein in your arm for cholesterol measurement. Some practices ask you to attend in the morning, having fasted overnight.

As heart attacks and coronary heart disease in general are very common in Britain, we must tackle the problem

The blood sample taken will then be tested for cholesterol, triglyceride and HDL cholesterol.

You can take the initiative

If your general practice is not running such a scheme and you feel that your blood cholesterol should be measured because you have a family history of coronary disease or a relative with a high cholesterol level, your doctor will be glad to do the blood tests. This is, however, only worthwhile if you are fully motivated to take any advice you are given, for example on diet or weight loss.

Different levels and what they mean

From the point of view of reducing the risk of a heart attack, it seems that the lower your blood cholesterol the better. To that end, most experts now recommend that all adults should at least adopt the eating habits discussed later in this book.

Such an approach, however, is not enough to help those people who start with relatively high cholesterol levels. Take, for example, a man whose cholesterol level is 8 mmol/l (the average is 5.7 mmol/l but even this is too high); supposing he were to reduce it by 20 per cent, which is not easily done, he would still have an undesirable level of 6.4 mmol/l; and in practice a 10 per cent reduction may be as much as he can achieve. Yet one adult in 25 in Britain has a cholesterol level of 8 mmol/l or more. In the same way, someone with a level of 6.5 mmol/l – and a quarter of us have levels of 6.5 or greater – will achieve a desirable level only if they reduce their cholesterol by 20 per cent or more.

CHOLESTEROL LEVELS

Mildly raised cholesterol level

If your cholesterol level is more than 5.2 mmol/l, your doctor will advise a cholesterol-lowering diet, and weight reduction if you are overweight. This is advice that all of us should follow, but there are important differences:

- Our motivation to eat healthily is greater if we know that we have a high cholesterol level and therefore an increased chance of having a heart attack.
- Our dieting efforts will be supervised by our doctor, a suitable diet sheet will be provided and there will be an explanation of why it is necessary.
- If your cholesterol is raised, and especially if there are other heart attack risk factors as well, your doctor or nurse may ask you to return for a further cholesterol test.

Very high blood cholesterol

If your cholesterol level is very high, the role of your doctor is greater. What to expect:

- Your treatment will start in the same way, by diet and, if needed, weight reduction.
- Regular repeat measurements, however, will be essential to ensure that the treatment is working.
- Your doctor will also see if there are other health problems that could give rise to a high cholesterol level, for example a lack of thyroid hormone or diabetes.
- Some drugs can also increase your blood cholesterol, so your doctor may choose to replace any you are taking with a safer alternative.
- Your doctor may refer you to a specialist at a hospital lipid clinic.

Guidelines on treatment

For people with high blood cholesterol levels, some medical guidance or treatment is often the only way of ensuring that satisfactory levels will be achieved. A panel of medical experts from 19 European countries has recently produced guidelines on how high blood cholesterol levels should be treated. They recommend that a health check to identify people at risk of heart attack should be available to all adults, and that it should include a blood cholesterol test. (The other information obtained in the health check should show how common coronary disease is in the person's close family and their smoking habits, body weight and blood pressure.)

If at first you don't succeed

If your cholesterol level does not fall enough, you could try a stricter cholesterol-lowering diet, under the close supervision of a dietician. Or your doctor may refer you to a special lipid clinic, of which there are now about 80 in Britain. But if thorough attempts fail to control the high cholesterol level through diet, it might be decided that you need the help of an anti-cholesterol drug in addition to the diet.

Screening the family

Another step that may be advised is for your close relatives – brothers and sisters, parents and children – to have cholesterol tests. This can be of help in two ways. First, we have seen that inheritance plays a role in most people with very high cholesterol levels, and so it may be helpful to the relatives of such people to be checked. Secondly, the pattern of inheritance may help the doctor to make an exact diagnosis.

Is it safe to lower blood cholesterol?

All medical treatments must be kept under continual scrutiny to ensure their safety. On the other hand, unjustified fears about a treatment could deprive people of care from which they would benefit. What do we know about the safety of lowered cholesterol levels?

- In countries such as Japan and Italy, where average blood cholesterol levels are (or used to be) low because the national diets were low in saturated fat, the average life span is longer than in countries such as Britain or the USA.
- Among groups of people, coronary death rates are highest in those groups in which cholesterol levels are highest. Some people with very low cholesterol levels (4 mmol/l or less, compared with the target level of 5.2 mmol/l) have an

increased risk of death from other causes.

However, when cholesterol is measured in young healthy working people, those with the lowest cholesterol levels have the least chance of dying, and the lowest risk of both coronary heart disease and of non-cardiac diseases such as cancer.

Sometimes, the link with low blood cholesterol appears to be due to a number of diseases which cause cholesterol levels to fall; for example, cancer cells produce cholesterol-lowering substances. But there are also a few unfortunate people who are, for unknown reasons, at increased risk of accidents and of serious chest problems, and also tend to have low cholesterol levels. However, there is no reason to believe that a low blood cholesterol level can *cause* non-cardiac disease.

- About 30 trials of cholesterol lowering have been carried out. These show that heart attacks are reduced, but do not tell us as much as we would like about effects on other illnesses. This is mostly because other serious illnesses are rare compared with heart attacks. In some trials, a non-cardiac illness occurred more commonly in those receiving treatment; in other trials, less commonly. Scientists have tried to see if these differences are due to anything more than random variation. The rates of cancer have, of course, been carefully scrutinized and the trials have shown no consistently favourable or unfavourable effect.

In three large trials of currently used cholesterol-lowering drugs, cancer rates were unaffected by treatment; and this was also the case in a third recent trial in which a very large reduction in cholesterol was achieved for 10 years.

In two out of the three recent trials there were more suicides and violent deaths among those who were assigned to the treatment groups. However, scientists working for an official body in the USA, the Food and Drugs Administration, have checked the case records of these fatalities. They found that many who had died accidental deaths or committed suicide had stopped taking their treatment years before. They also found that some of the accidents seemed unavoidable, as was the case with those treated subjects who were the victims of suicide. The scientists' conclusion was that there was no evidence that lowering blood cholesterol, or the cholesterol-lowering drugs themselves, had led to an increase in deaths from these causes.

In the most recent large trial, in men with pre-existing heart disease, those who received a powerful cholesterol-lowering drug had fewer recurrences of heart disease, *and also fewer deaths from all causes – in other words they lived longer.*

Some drugs, used in early trials of coronary prevention, proved to have toxic effects. They included massive doses of certain hormones. Their influence on blood cholesterol levels was small, and the harmful effects were due to other actions, probably on heart rhythm and on blood clotting. Such drugs are of course no longer used.

Those trials in which the fall in blood cholesterol was greatest (15 to 23 per cent) usually show a reduction in total death rates; if cholesterol lowering were harmful, such trials would be expected to show an increase in mortality.

What is the balance of evidence?

The evidence that heart attack rates are reduced by lowering high blood cholesterol is now overwhelmingly strong. By contrast, there is no convincing evidence that lowering cholesterol causes serious diseases or accidents.

So it would be wrong to forego the benefits of a healthier diet, or of medically prescribed treatments, because of unsupported concerns about safety.

Treating a high cholesterol level

Effective treatment is now available for almost everyone who has a high cholesterol level, and, to some extent, this has been discussed in earlier chapters. A change in diet is the only treatment needed for most people with high blood cholesterol; but for adults who have inherited familial hypercholesterolaemia or other major genetic problems it is also usually necessary for the doctor to prescribe one, occasionally two, drugs in order to bring the cholesterol levels down to safe target values. There is a third group whose high cholesterol levels are not definitely caused by a major inherited disorder but who, nevertheless, fail to respond adequately to diet. They may also sometimes need to receive drug treatment if the doctor decides that they are at serious risk of heart trouble. Drugs are never a substitute for careful attention to diet,

and the doctor will usually only consider a drug if repeated dietary efforts to achieve target levels over a period of about a year have failed.

How much treatment is needed?

When should a raised cholesterol level be treated vigorously and when are milder measures appropriate? Can high cholesterol levels safely be ignored in some circumstances?

The answers depend on one's overall risk of having a heart attack. This is influenced by the many factors referred to in earlier parts of this book, and we now look at their joint influence by asking some basic questions.

- Do you already have coronary disease – that is, have you had a heart attack, do you have angina, or have you had an operation on your coronary arteries? Or do you have arterial trouble in your legs? If the answer to any of these is 'yes', your doctor will usually advise careful treatment of all risk factors and a raised cholesterol level will, as a rule, be vigorously treated. Even mildly raised levels should be dealt with.

- Has a parent, brother or sister developed coronary disease before age 60, or has this happened in a number of more distant blood relatives? Such a family history contributes to your overall risk and justifies more active treatment.

- Do you smoke cigarettes, or were you a heavy smoker until recently?

- Has a doctor diagnosed you as having diabetes or high blood pressure?

- Has a doctor diagnosed you as having an inherited form of high blood cholesterol, such as familial hypercholesterolaemia or remnant hyperlipidaemia?

If the answer to one or more of these questions is 'yes', the treatment of high cholesterol levels will be more vigorous.

Until late in life, coronary disease is commoner in men than in women. In young women the problem is rare, although this trend changes after the menopause.

Before the change of life, most women with high cholesterol levels will receive dietary advice; only those who have an inherited form, and those at higher risk because of smoking or diabetes, for example, may need drug treatment.

Views on the influence of age have changed. A high level of cholesterol continues to increase risk at least into the 70s, and most heart attacks occur after age 60. Advancing age is often a justification for vigorous treatment rather than the reverse, except in the very old.

As the different lipoproteins (especially LDL and HDL) have opposite effects on risk, your doctor will usually want to be informed about the balance between these substances before treating a high blood cholesterol level with a drug. A high level of LDL means increased risk. The risk is even greater if the HDL level is low, whereas a moderately high level of LDL is less of a problem if the HDL is also high.

Quite commonly in older people, HDL levels are remarkably high, and this can lead to a moderately raised blood cholesterol level. If the LDL is normal, such a person is at low risk and does not require any treatment. This condition is especially common in women receiving hormone replacement therapy (HRT) after the menopause; it can also occur in people who are young, slim and athletic.

One last point: having more than one risk factor has a greater effect on risk than might be expected. Just a few cigarettes per day, together with a mildly raised blood pressure, increases the risk quite a lot. Removing both of these risk factors, which can be done quite easily, will have a large effect in reducing risk.

Diet depends on body weight

The diet your doctor will advise will depend on whether you are overweight or lean, and he will check your weight and height against a chart to decide if you need to lose weight.

If you have high blood cholesterol levels, he may recommend the sort of diet set out in the next few pages. Such a diet also helps to lower high triglyceride (fat) levels in the blood.

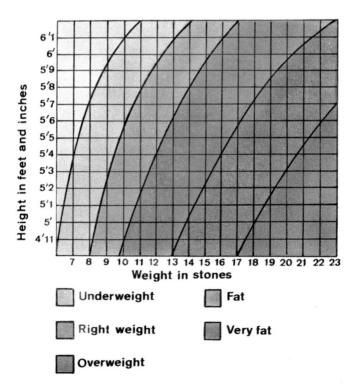

Chart relating weight and height to obesity.

Cholesterol-lowering diet for lean people

Choose freely from the list of suitable foods. You may have a moderate portion of items in the limited foods list once a week. The foods to be avoided are self-explanatory and, if eaten at all, their use should be very rare. The diet is based on the principles explained on pages 24 – 27.

Breakfast

Suitable

Oatmeal (such as porridge or muesli) or other whole-grain cereal with skimmed milk
Wholemeal bread or crispbread with soft margarine high in polyunsaturates and/or marmalade, jam, yeast extract or skimmed-milk cheese (such as cottage cheese, quark, fromage frais labelled 0% fat)
Haddock
Very low fat yoghurt
Fruit – fresh, dried or stewed
Coffee, tea

Limited

Refined breakfast cereal
White bread, bread baked with egg
Kippers, smoked salmon, fish paste
Very lean grilled bacon
Semi-skimmed milk

Avoid

Cereals containing coconut, sugar-frosted cereals
Butter
Whole milk, cream

Lunch and dinner

Suitable

Clear soup, home-made vegetable soup, broth
Any fish (white or oily)
Veal, turkey or chicken (without skin)
Game, rabbit, hare
Pulses, such as lentils, kidney beans, butter beans, haricot beans, mung beans, chick peas
Root vegetables, salads, leafy vegetables
Plain or wholemeal pastas, boiled rice (preferably brown) or potatoes
Spices, herbs (avoid added salt), low-fat salad cream, specified oils (see page 50)
Fruit (have at least three pieces per day, one or more of which should be citrus)
Low-fat fruit sorbet, very-low-fat yoghurt

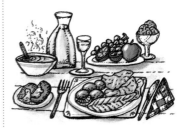

Matzo, water biscuits, wholemeal bread with soft margarine high in polyunsaturates
Walnuts, chestnuts
Coffee, tea, mineral water, wine (see *Alcoholic drinks* on pages 45 and 50)

Limited

Packet or canned soups
Very lean beef, spring lamb, pork or pork products
Whole egg (two each week, but egg white is not restricted)
Liver (every 2 weeks)
Mussels, oysters, other shellfish (every 2 to 4 weeks)
Avocados
Low-fat hard cheeses

Avoid

All fatty meat and meat products (fat may be visible on the meat, or hidden as in sausages, paté, pies), duck, goose, minced meat (unless prepared from very lean beef)
Roe, including caviar and taramasalata
Egg pastas
Sweetbreads, tongue, brain, kidney
Foods fried or roasted in oils or fats not on specified list (see page 50) or unknown
Potato crisps, coconut, cashew nuts
Ice cream, prepared puddings
Pastries, cakes, biscuits (unless baked with oils or fats on specified list, see page 50)
Whole milk, cream, butter, full-fat cheese

Coffee and tea time snacks

Suitable

Crispbread, wholemeal bread or toast, matzo (not egg matzo)
Cake, biscuits, oatcakes baked with suitable fat (page 50)
Tea, coffee, unsweetened fruit juice,

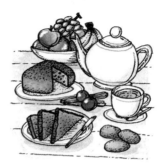

sugar-free soft drinks, mineral water
Snacks comprising raw vegetables
Fruit, dried fruits

Limited

Marzipan, halva, Turkish delight, boiled sweets

Avoid

Cakes and other foods baked with fat not on specified list (see page 50) or unknown
Deep-fried snacks
Chocolates, toffees, fudge, most confectionery bars
Coffee whitener made with palm oil
Peanut butter
Foods containing coconut fat or palm oil

Cholesterol-lowering, weight-reducing diet for overweight people

Getting rid of excess pounds (or stones) is especially important for people with high cholesterol levels, and eating fewer calories is the priority until your target weight is achieved. Your doctor will provide you with a reducing diet if necessary, and it will have much in common with the cholesterol-lowering diet for lean people. Ideally you will lose about one to two pounds (half to one kilogram) each week.

A limited list of very low-calorie foods

Only a small number of foods which contain very few calories (when consumed in ordinary amounts) can be eaten freely. They include, for example:
Clear soups and broths
Most salad vegetables (except avocados)
Leafy vegetables
Asparagus
Grapefruit
Rhubarb
Unsweetened black tea and coffee
Sugar-free soft drinks and mineral waters

About the diet

The diet provides daily allowances of other permitted foods, the amount depending on how much exercise and physical work you do and how big you are. The following diet is an example, but only your doctor or dietician can specify your personal requirements. If you are more than mildly overweight, you should be supervised by a doctor and/or a dietician.

Breakfast

One slice wholemeal bread (30 g, 1 oz) or two crispbreads or sugar-free high-fibre breakfast cereal
Marmite or Bovril or fish paste
Unsaturated margarine small amount
Skimmed milk
Half a grapefruit
Lean grilled bacon or ham (30 g, 1 oz) twice weekly
Tea or coffee with skimmed milk and permitted sweetener

11.00 am

Tea or coffee with skimmed milk and permitted sweetener

Lunch

Clear soup or home-made vegetable soup
Very low-fat cottage cheese (140 g, 5 oz) or grilled, steamed or baked fish (140 g, 5 oz)

or grilled very lean meat (55 g, 2 oz) or boiled egg (from allowance)
Green vegetables, salad vegetables, asparagus, cauliflower, mushrooms
Small helping of French beans, broad beans, peas, artichoke or carrots
One crispbread
Unsaturated margarine: small amount
One or two pieces of fruit e.g. apple, orange, plum or half banana

4.00 pm

Tea or coffee with skimmed milk and permitted sweetener
Two crispbreads
or one slice wholemeal bread (30 g, 1 oz)
Marmite, Bovril or fish paste

Dinner

As lunch

10.00 pm

Tea with skimmed milk or lemon and permitted sweetener

Permitted items as snacks

Clear soup or soup made from bouillon cube
Fresh vegetables, for example asparagus, carrot, cauliflower, celery, cucumber, lettuce, mushrooms
Half grapefruit, gooseberries
One or two other pieces of fruit

Daily allowances

Polyunsaturated margarine (20 g, 2/3 oz)
Skimmed milk (270 ml, half a pint) or milk made from dried skimmed milk powder (30 g, 1 oz)
Very-low-fat cottage cheese (140 g, 5 oz)
or fish (140 g, 5 oz)
or very lean meat (55 g, 2 oz)
Eggs – up to two per week

Please avoid

Unfortunately there is quite a long list of foods that must be avoided entirely until you reach your target weight, and they will have to be eaten or drunk rather sparingly indefinitely if you are to maintain that weight and keep your cholesterol low. These include:

- Fatty meat and poultry such as duck
- Cream, butter, whole milk, cheese
- Fried foods
- Alcohol
- Sugar, jams, honey, chocolates, sweets, sugar-containing drinks
- Cakes, biscuits

Regular, suitable aerobic exercise will also help you to lose weight. Aim for at least three hours per week of mild to moderate activity. If you are very overweight, or if you have high overall risk of coronary disease, consult your doctor before starting any exercise programme.

Alcoholic drinks

Although alcohol does not directly increase the level of blood cholesterol, it is a common cause of high blood fat (triglyceride) levels.

As a concentrated source of calories and (often) an appetite stimulant, it is an important cause of obesity.

Alcohol is a significant cause of raised blood pressure too, especially, but not only, If drunk in large amounts by susceptible people. Of course, heavy drinkers are also prone to disease of the liver, brain, nerves, muscles and other organs. Despite all these problems, alcoholic drinks are one of life's pleasures and, used in moderation, alcohol seems to be harmless to most of us.

What is moderation? Well, one to three drinks per day are harmless to most men, and one to two are acceptable for most women (unless they are overweight). One drink is defined as a half-pint of an average beer, a single tot of spirits, a wine glass of an unfortified table wine or a sherry glass of sherry, port or Madeira.

Some recent research has shown that people who have two or three drinks a day have a lower rate of heart disease than people who drink more or less than this.

Alcohol tolerance is greater in men than in women, at least so far as liver disease is concerned.

Oils and fats

As discussed earlier, the type and amount of fat in the diet are the main external factors controlling blood cholesterol levels.

These have been taken into account in designing the diet suggestions listed above. Large amounts of any oil or fat are best avoided. Suitable oils include sunflower, olive, corn, walnut and soybean.

It will also be helpful if you get into the habit of reading the nutritional information panel on food packages. The government and voluntary bodies are actively working on ways of improving food labelling.

Beware of foods that carry vague information such as 'contains no animal fat' or 'contains pure vegetable oil'.

DRUG TREATMENT OF HIGH BLOOD CHOLESTEROL

Doctors now have a wide range of effective, safe drugs for lowering raised cholesterol levels. But it cannot be said too often that the first approach to treatment of high blood cholesterol is by diet. This may also be true of the treatment of mildly – and moderately – high blood pressure, although currently the emphasis in blood pressure treatment is on drugs rather than diet. With high blood cholesterol, on the other hand, you will be treated by diet at first and only if this persistently fails will the combination of diet and drug treatment be introduced.

Remember too that drug treatment for cholesterol problems has to be continued indefinitely, as with treatment for high blood pressure or diabetes. Here are some of the drugs your doctor may consider.

Resins

The two in this group are cholestyramine (Questran) or colestipol (Colestid); these drugs lower cholesterol levels by increasing the breakdown of LDL in the liver. The redundant cholesterol is converted into bile acids in the liver, and these are excreted from the body, bound to the drug (which is itself completely excreted). None of the drug is absorbed into the body, which is an important safety feature.

Both these drugs are provided in powder form and have to be taken at mealtimes in quite large quantities, suspended in fruit juice or water.

Drugs that suppress cholesterol production

The names of these drugs end in '-statin'. They are much more recent than resins and three are now licensed for use in Britain: fluvastatin (Lescol), pravastatin (Lipostat) and simvastatin (Zocor). They are exceedingly effective, and usually a single dose is taken each evening. They are the most potent cholesterol-lowering drugs now available (and taken with a resin they offer the best treatment for people with very high levels). A controlled trial has shown both a reduction in heart disease and a good safety record.

Fibrates

Several drugs fall into this group, and have the letters '...fibr...' in their names. They reduce triglyceride (fat) levels most effectively, but also lower cholesterol. In addition, they increase the level of HDL cholesterol, which may prove to help protect against heart attack. They also reduce levels of the clotting factor called fibrinogen, another possible source of benefit. Gemfibrozil (Lopid) and clofibrate (Atromid) have been shown to reduce the risk of coronary disease, but clofibrate is no longer widely used because it can increase the chance of developing gallstones. New drugs in this category seem to be very effective.

Other lipid-lowering drugs

There are other lipid-lowering drugs that have particular uses, but at present are less widely prescribed.

A word about regular check-ups

If your doctor treats you with a cholesterol-lowering drug he will need to see you repeatedly to confirm its effectiveness and to ask you about side effects. Some blood tests are also useful in checking for side effects. Should you be treated by diet, your doctor may also want to check that you have responded; this is necessary after two to four months if your level was substantially high (over 6.5 mmol/l) but not usually if you only had a marginally high level (5.2 to 6.5 mmol/l). If no active treatment is given it is good practice to repeat the cholesterol test, and check other risk factors every five years.

OTHER TREATMENTS

Regular exercise

We have already seen that many research findings suggest that regular exercise may help protect against heart attack. The kind and amount of exercise must be tailored to your age, your level of physical fitness and whether you have any diseases of the heart, lungs, joints and muscles; otherwise minor injuries or, occasionally, major problems may result. If you are in middle age or older and are unfit it is wise to have a medical check-up *before* taking up exercise, and you must start with light exercise, increasing gradually over several months as your fitness improves.

Exercise should be reasonably frequent (three to four times weekly) and the length of time spent exercising is more important in preventing heart problems than the intensity of exercise. Starting with a few minutes at a time you should gradually progress to periods of 20 to 40 minutes. If in any doubt, it is best to have your exercise programme supervised, for example at a well-run gym. The most suitable forms of exercise are those that increase the pumping action of the heart, such as fast walking, jogging, swimming, light calisthenics or aerobics and vigorous dancing. Although ball games may be more pleasurable, the level of exercise is not under your control and can become excessive if you are in middle age or older.

Avoiding cholesterol-raising drugs

Some drugs widely used in the treatment of high blood pressure and certain skin conditions, including acne, can raise cholesterol and triglyceride levels. If your blood cholesterol is high, your doctor will consider the pros and cons of replacing such a drug by one that does not increase the cholesterol.

Some drugs lower cholesterol: the use of female hormone (oestrogen) in hormone replacement therapy (HRT) at the time of the menopause often reduces levels of cholesterol and LDL and increases HDL.

Rarely needed treatments

Very rarely indeed a patient is seen whose cholesterol level is extremely high and particularly resistant to diet and drug treatment. Such people have usually inherited a gene for familial hypercholesterolaemia from each parent. The high cholesterol level (sometimes as much as 20 mmol/l) may show itself as yellowish deposits in the skin during childhood.

This used to be a serious and untreatable problem with heart disease developing in adolescence. Now, due to a technique pioneered at the Hammersmith Hospital in London, cholesterol levels can be dramatically lowered by a combination of drugs and a procedure called LDL-apheresis. In LDL-apheresis, the patient's blood is passed through an instrument that absorbs most of the LDL from it. This has to be repeated every one to three weeks indefinitely.

A more recent, equally dramatic, advance in treatment of this rare disease is liver transplantation, although this is still in an experimental stage.

In summary

WHAT CAN YOU DO?

The steps that you can take to avoid coronary disease are supported by extensive research, so that there is reasonable certainty about the benefits of the first three below and a fair probability about the last two:

- do not smoke;
- avoid becoming overweight and reduce weight if you need to;
- choose the kinds of food recommended (on pages 46–47);
- take regular exercise of a type and amount suitable for your age and state of fitness and health;
- learn and use techniques for relaxing and for coping with stress.

This book is written for healthy people who want to lessen the chances of suffering from coronary disease and other illnesses affecting the circulation. It is also for people who already have coronary problems, because reducing cholesterol and other risk factors is an important aspect of their treatment.

THE CENTRAL ROLE OF CHOLESTEROL

The main topic of this book is the role of cholesterol in coronary disease. This illness has many causes, but one very important cause is a high level of cholesterol in the blood. Other causes do not seem to lead to much coronary disease unless the diet, and the resultant blood cholesterol, are unsatisfactory.

INHERITING THE RISK

In addition to the influence of diet, blood cholesterol is strongly affected by inheritance. This is one of the reasons why heart attacks tend to run in families. Even the very high levels of cholesterol that can be inherited can be effectively reduced by diet and, if necessary, by safe but powerful drugs.

So, it is important that these disorders are detected early in life to provide the best chance of avoiding heart trouble.

TAKE RESPONSIBILITY FOR YOUR HEALTH

Preventing illness always depends on a joint effort between you and your doctor.

Now you have read this book you will understand how you can play your part in helping to avoid heart trouble.

Useful Addresses

British Heart Foundation
14 Fitzhardinge Street, London W1H
4DH Tel: (0171) 935 0185
  Wide range of publications, leaflets
  and local groups

Family Heart Association
Wesley House, 7 High Street,
Kidlington, Oxford OX5 2DH
  Tel: (01865) 370292
  Literature for GPs and patients, free
  loan of cholesterol testing
  equipment to GPs, 24-hour
  cholesterol and diet helpline,
  medical and nutritional advice
  about lipids.

Index